O P E N
B O D Y

Creating Your Own Yoga

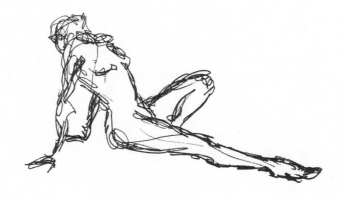

TODD WALTON
with drawings by Vance Lawry

AVON BOOKS 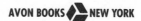 NEW YORK

Excerpt from *Ida Rolf Talks About Rolfing and Physical Reality*
edited by Rosemary Feitis, a Harper Colophon Book,
published in 1978.

AVON BOOKS
a division of
The Hearst Corporation
1350 Avenue of the Americas
New York, New York 10019

Copyright © 1998 by Todd Walton
Artwork © 1998 by Vance Lawry
Interior design by the author
Published by arrangement with the author
Visit our website at http://www.AvonBooks.com
Library of Congress Catalog Card Number: 98-92426
ISBN: 0-380-79535-3

First Avon Books Trade Printing: May 1998

AVON TRADEMARK REG. U.S. PAT. OFF. AND IN OTHER COUNTRIES,
MARCA REGISTRADA, HECHO EN U.S.A.

Printed in the U.S.A.

QPH 10 9 8 7 6 5 4 3 2 1

for my mother who encouraged me to dance and sing,
for my father who challenged me to tell the truth,
and in loving memory of Susan Marcia Keusch,
who touched so many people's lives,
guiding them on a path to inner peace.
May she have found her own—
so richly deserved.

So many people are still asking,
What should I feel?
I say to them, Well, who the heck knows what
you should feel except you?
I can't feel what you feel.
It's very important, with some people,
to shift their attention and get their agreement
to take responsibility for themselves.

Ida Rolf

Contents

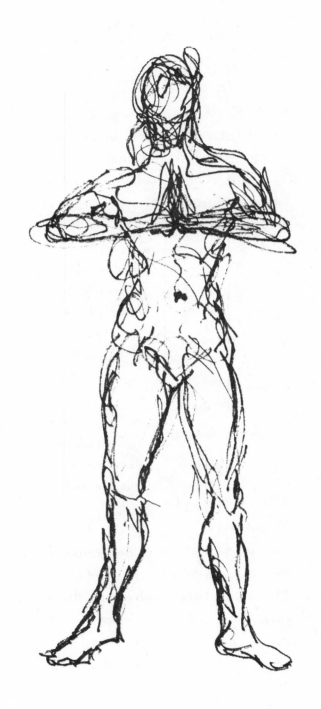

Welcome

Whether you are conscious of it or not, your life is an act of indivisible cooperation between your mind and your body. Perhaps you chose to look into this book because the ideas conveyed by the words on the cover aroused your curiosity. Or perhaps you reached for it reflexively, responding to a directive—obvious or subtle—from your body.

Humans are innately curious. Our success, both as individuals and as a species, is largely the result of our indefatigable desire to explore that which intrigues us. Your curiosity about your body is a wonderful sign of your desire to know more about yourself, and to heal further.

Have no fear. You need know nothing about yoga to understand and enjoy this book. The ideas contained herein will complement any book or course of study focusing on physical fitness, yoga, or the care and maintenance of your body.

For anyone suffering from pain and tension, either physical or emotional, and for those of you intent on improving your flexibility and strength, this book should prove helpful and thought-provoking.

Welcome.

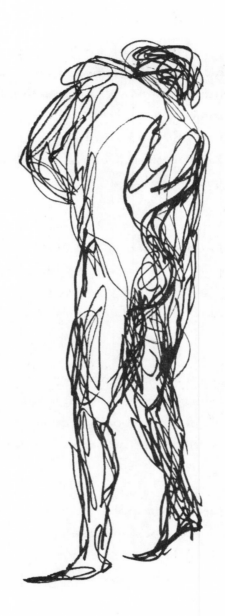

Why

I have written this book to help you overcome your fears and misconceptions about yoga, and to ignite your creative responses to your body.

Many people feel intimidated by yoga books and magazines featuring extremely limber practitioners demonstrating various yoga postures. Even people who have had excellent instructors often compare themselves to more supple students. They may cease their practice because they feel inferior, or because they've hurt themselves trying to do more than their bodies are ready to do.

I have struggled for much of my life with extreme stiffness, pain, and immobility. I began practicing yoga when I was eighteen, having exhausted all standard medical approaches for treating a condition diagnosed as advanced ankylosing spondylitis, which is derived from the Greek "agkulos" meaning to "crook". Put simply, it is a premature stiffening and eventual fusing of vertebrae and joints.

I will never forget the swift onset of my pain. I was fifteen years old. I woke on a Monday morning, aching from head to toe, having played a bone-crunching game of tackle football the day before. To my relief, the soreness wore off after I walked the mile to school. However, when I woke on Tuesday morning, I could barely move my legs. Fierce, shooting pains raced through my lower back and hips. Feeling somewhat better after a hot shower, I took three aspirin and walked to school. Again, most of the soreness left me. But on Wednesday morning, there was no getting out of bed. I was completely paralyzed with pain.

And so began a grueling ordeal of examinations by medical specialists, along with countless x-rays and blood tests to determine what was wrong with me. When my condition was finally diagnosed, I began taking powerful anti-inflammatory drugs that did little to alleviate my pain and left me deeply depressed.

Three years later, when I moved out of my parents' house to attend college, I vowed to stop using all prescription painkillers and anti-inflammatory drugs. I wanted to find ways to cope with my pain and immobility that did not dampen my spirit. With only aspirin and warm showers to aid me, I was often incapable of moving without killing pain. I missed classes and distressed my friends, but I was determined to find a natural way to live with my disability. I experienced passages of time where I was fairly mobile, but inevitably the pain would gather force and fell me again.

Then one day, intrigued by a course description in my college catalogue, I signed up for a yoga class. On the morning of the first session, I hobbled down to the gymnasium and peered into a room bursting with limber young women in colorful leotards. They were all stretching and bending their bodies in ways I couldn't imagine ever bending or stretching mine. Deeply embarrassed to be the only male present, I barely stayed long enough to get a five-page hand-out describing a dozen basic yoga postures, illustrated with drawings of incredibly flexible women.

Feeling too stiff and unattractive to expose my physical limitations in the company of such elastic bodies, I dropped the yoga class and began practicing the postures alone in my room. Slowly but surely, I began to feel a little looser, a little more comfortable in my body.

To learn more about what I was doing, I acquired copies of the few yoga books available in 1967, and though I continued to feel intimidated by the ideal bodies of advanced practitioners, my need was great so I persevered.

After working every day for a year to improve my flexibility, and feeling quite proud of my progress, I introduced a friend to yoga. With his first attempts at the basic postures, he surpassed all my efforts with ease.

I became very discouraged, discontinued my practice for the next few months, and experienced a debilitating increase in pain. When I became so incapacitated I could barely walk, I finally bid farewell to my wounded pride and resumed my yoga. Within a few days, my pain decreased dramatically and I felt loose enough to play a little Frisbee. This was the turning point in my relationship to yoga, and the beginning of my modifications to formal approaches.

My yoga was not the yoga of my friend. My yoga was not the yoga of the lithe person in the how-to book. My yoga was, and remains after thirty years, my personal response to the needs of *my* body.

I hope this book will enhance your relationship to your most miraculous creation—you.

Now

No two bodies are alike. This is a scientific fact. Yours is not the body in the how-to book. You don't look or feel like anyone else. At the beginning, and in the end, your body is unique.

By the same token, no two body pains are alike. Her back pain is not his, nor is yours mine. Every pain is specific to the body that holds it.

It is my belief that we each practice a personal yoga through which our body forms itself. For instance, how are you standing or sitting at this moment? This "reading position" is probably one of your basic postures. You have chosen it for both comfort and balance.

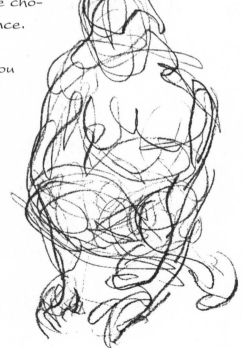

Take a minute to examine how you are holding yourself. Do you find that you favor one side of your body over the other? Can you imagine this pose creating an imbalance in your strength or flexibility? Try assuming the mirror-opposite position. How does that make your body feel?

Most of us close as we age, physically and emotionally. Our

shoulders curl in over our hearts. We begin to mistrust people older or younger than ourselves. We become narrow-minded and wary of change. We hold ourselves stiffly. Pain sets in. But we don't have to close as we age. We can use our personal yoga to become more open than ever before.

Think of something quite simple
that you always do the same way—
putting on your socks, for example.
Try to do it a completely
different way, without
hurting yourself,
of course. I think
you'll find that varying a
routine action can be
extremely revealing about
how our physical choices
define us.

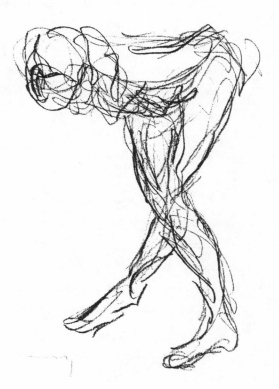

Definitions

Yoga is a Sanskrit word meaning
the union of the physical self with the universal spirit

In the Hindu and Buddhist traditions, yoga encompasses various aspects of existence: physical, mental, emotional, and spiritual. There are vast texts and ancient lineages representing myriad schools of yogic teachings. About these matters, I am the most fledgling of students.

I use the word "yoga" to mean all those physical and verbal and emotional and meditative things I do in loving response to the needs of my body and spirit.

Yoga might be breathing slowly to calm yourself, to help you focus on a single issue.

Yoga might be doing push-ups with an intention to strengthen your body.

Yoga might be seventeen postures from the ancient texts of "asana" and "pranayama."

Yoga might be different ways of lying in bed.

Yoga might be humming with a friend.

Yoga might be seven variations on a smile.

Yoga might be the dance you do while washing the dishes.

My grandmother Goody, who possessed the energy of a healthy child for all of her eighty years, practiced a personal yoga she called her "feel-good regimen." She went on twice-daily walks that took her all around the town she lived in. Over the years, she became extremely familiar with the people and animals and gardens along her way. She not only stretched her body when she walked, she helped create community.

Goody also sang every day, swung her arms, touched her toes, did facial stretches, and danced whenever the music suited her fancy. Her meditation practice involved a daily reading of the *Bible*. She would read from *Psalms*, then close her eyes to ponder the words.

What are some of your activities that invigorate and relax you? You might want to make a list of them under the heading *My Yoga*. Honoring your physical choices in this way will almost certainly give them new meaning and power.

Who are you?

And speaking of definitions, how do you define yourself? It is my belief that our bodies hold the answer to this fundamental question. If you want to heal yourself, it is extremely helpful to know who it is you're healing. Indeed, it has been my experience that physical discomfort, illness, and even injury often go hand in hand with a conflicted self-image or an unresolved feeling about myself.

Sit comfortably and take a few quiet moments to think about your parents. Can you see their faces, their bodies? These are your progenitors, the beings to whom the blueprint of your body was entrusted. Do you see parts of yourself—postures, gestures, attitudes—in them? Any you want to let go of?

Close your eyes and conjure an image of yourself when you were younger. Wait until you have a clear memory of yourself. Now open your chest, gently pulling your shoulders back as far as you can without causing pain. Hold yourself open and take a deep breath, imagining the air to be a breathable form of love. As you exhale, send this love out into the world.

To take this process further, stand comfortably and extend your arms out from your side. With palms facing forward, press your hands back into the emptiness behind you, breathing slowly and deeply. As you hold

yourself open, ask aloud, "Who am I?" Now answer
with whatever words come into your mind. Try not to
censor yourself, for even if what you say seems
nonsensical or simplistic or unpleasant,
your spontaneous answer will very
likely provide you with
valuable food for thought.

Intention

Intention is a fundamental concern of all spiritual practices, and is particularly important in yoga and meditation.

What do you intend to do? Climb a mountain? Meditate for ten minutes? Embrace a loved one?

What is at the center of your focus?
What is motivating you?

Is your intention joyful? Loving? Fierce?
Fiercely loving?

Yoga masters believe that
the quality of our
intention influences our
ability to expand and heal
as profoundly as the
physical practice itself.

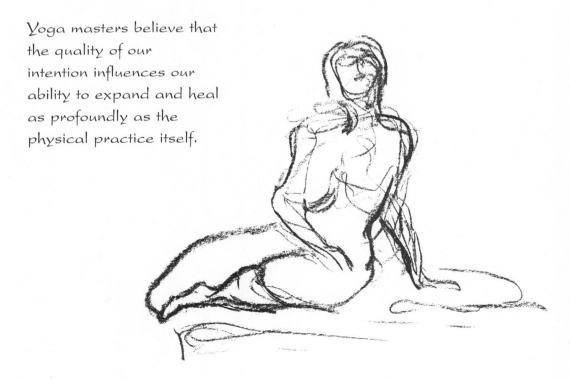

Intention is closely related to Attention. When your intention is clear, it is easier to pay attention.

Paying attention is all about being fully present—free of the past and the future.

Sit or stand comfortably in good light and carefully examine a small natural object—a stone or a leaf or a feather. Allow this object to entirely fill your vision. Now close your eyes, holding an image of the object in your mind. When the image begins to fade, open your eyes and examine the object again. Now close your eyes and relax. If you are not in the habit of examining tiny things, you may find this a helpful exercise for developing concentration and focus in other areas of your life.

That stretching sensation

Stretch your fingers. Wiggle your toes. Roll your shoulders. All our appendages are major energy conductors. If they are too tight, too closed, certain energies cannot gain release.

Stretch to expand, not to strain. When we strain, we override our body's ability to tell us how it feels about what we're trying to do. Put another way: Give it a try, but don't force it.

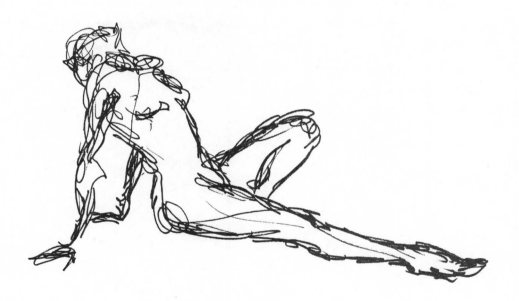

Even a little bit of stretching makes the body feel better. Too often we stop ourselves from giving our body any exercise because we think it needs a thorough and intensive workout for the exercise to be beneficial.

When my cat Tiny wakes from a nap, she stretches her legs out in front of her and raises her hindquarters high in the air. After holding this pose for a moment, she arches her back and yawns mightily. We are more like cats than you might suspect. We love feeling strong and stretched and easy in our bodies.

Sit on the edge of your bed and imagine that you are a cat waking from a nap. Stretch your arms toward the ceiling, stretching your fingers, too. Allow this gentle stretch to lift you to your feet and up onto your toes. Now lower your arms to your sides and stand comfortably. Lean to the left, now lean to the right. Roll your shoulders. Take a deep breath and exhale with an audible sound. Now—like any good cat— you're ready to go exploring.

What feels good to you?

Try lying on your back. Do this on a foam pad or on a firm bed. Use a pillow under your head if you need to. Shift around until you are most comfortable.

Lie still for several moments, remembering to breathe deeply. When you feel relaxed, hold your breath for as long as you can before exhaling.

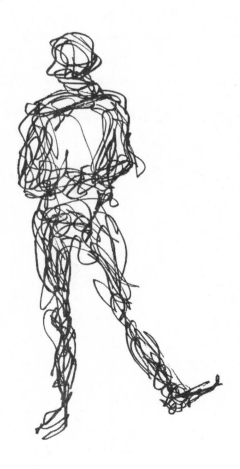

Imagine that your body is an egg, and that you are the baby bird inside. Wiggle around as if you are squirming to be born. You may wish to do this before you leave your bed in the morning or as a prelude to sleeping.

What feels good to you?

Lying still? Moving in slow motion? Dancing?
Taking a walk? Swimming? Singing?

Even if you don't feel you have much time to spare, choose something you enjoy, and do it.

Your body will appreciate any attention you give it.

Stretching through movement

Stand comfortably. Raise your right shoulder and, as you lower it, raise your left. As you lower your left shoulder, raise your right, alternating back and forth. This is the beginning of undulation—a very good loosening motion.

With or without music to accompany you, use this easy shoulder movement to lead your body into a gentle dance. Imagine your body undulating like a snake. Move your hands, arms, shoulders, legs, hips, back, and head in rhythm to your vision of undulation.

Move until you feel your-self growing warmer. Only your body can make this particular kind of heat. It is your personal antidote to tension and pain. Through your unique form of movement, you can free yourself of frozen energies.

Your movement, your dance, is the song of your body.

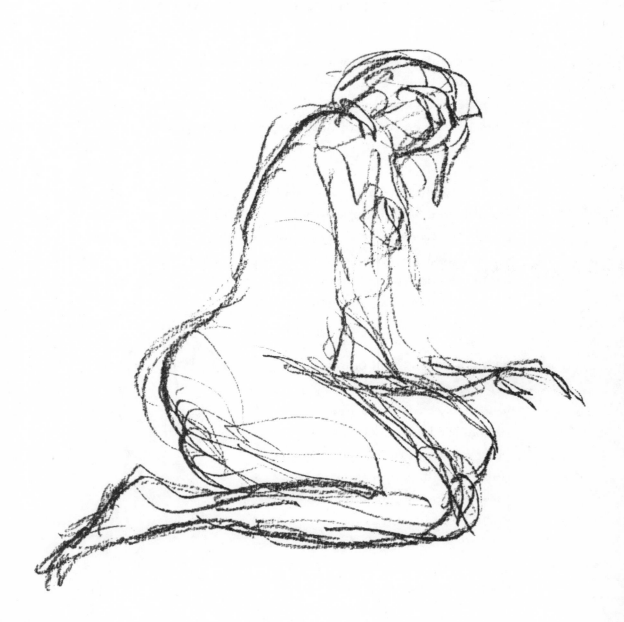

Finding your pains

Pain is an important part of our body's language. To become more fluent in this language, we must learn to be aware of subtle bodily sensations. By calming ourselves and listening to (sensing) the internal flow of signals, we can better decide how to move or stretch to relieve tension.

Stretching amplifies calls for attention from various parts of our bodies. Muscles sing as we stretch them. This singing is the release of previously compacted information. Does one pain call louder than the others? A loud pain is usually involved with more than one part of your body.

Stretch to enlarge the point of discomfort. For example, if your neck is stiff, cradle your chin in one hand and place your other hand on the back of your head. Now gently turn your head very slightly to one side. This may hurt a little, but don't let the pain stop your explorations. You are making room in a painful place for blood and lymph and oxygen—all of which are essential to healing. After you've stretched a painful place, give the area a gentle massage to further loosen things up.

Yoga seeks to give every part of the body an opportunity to express its state of openness, and to help you open further.

Appearance

I once suggested to a woman with chronic back pain that it might speed her healing if she would examine herself in a mirror, naked. If she felt displeased with any part of herself, I urged her to investigate the possible connection between her pain and those parts of herself she found objectionable.

She replied, "It's too much to ask of most women. We have so much shame about our bodies not being like the bodies in the fashion magazines."

Acknowledging this, and honoring every person's struggle to love her or his unique configuration of parts, I still wish for you to know your body as intimately as you possibly can. I believe that *every* body is the ideal body. To be told by anyone that our essential shape or size is wrong or bad is abusive to our soul and damaging to our well-being. It is a cultural disgrace that so much of our media propagandizes against all but a narrow spectrum of body types.

Are you as strong as you want to be? Are you limber enough to do all the things you would enjoy doing? Do you feel healthy and energetic? How do you—that remarkable intermingling of mind, body, and soul—feel? These are the important questions we can address through healthful effort.

Stand before a mirror, as clothed as you need to be.
Look at yourself, all of yourself. Breathe deeply and
relax. Imagine that your reflection is someone you're
meeting for the first time, someone fascinating and full
of surprises, someone worthy of your trust and
admiration. Now kiss your hands and watch your
reflection kiss its hands. Now kiss your reflection and
pour your love into this moving picture of the person
you wish to heal.

Run a hot bath. Soak. Open your chest. Hold it open
and allow the heat to penetrate you, to loosen you.
Relax. Now hold yourself open again and breathe
deeply, imagining your breath entering those newly
opened parts of yourself. Relax. Open again. Breathe
deeply. Think of this
warm immersion
as a gift to the
person you love.

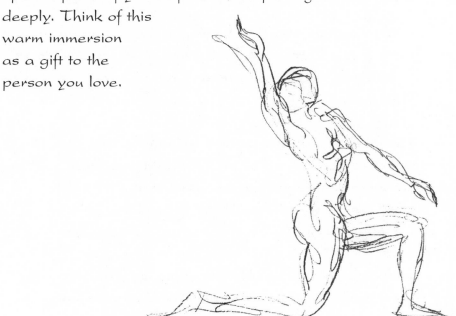

Bed yoga

There were times when I was in too much pain to do yoga on the floor, even on a thick mat, so I started doing stretches in bed. Now I do a bit of yoga in bed every day.

Remove your covers and lie on your back. Roll your head gently from side to side. How stiff is your neck today?

Spread your legs and stretch your toes. Make yourself as wide and expanded as you can. Relax. Expand. Relax.

Roll onto your stomach. Which cheek do you prefer resting on? Try them both. If you are uncomfortable, lift yourself up on your elbows and roll your head to loosen your neck.

Remaining on your stomach, grip the edges of your bed and pull yourself into the center of the mattress. Keeping your legs straight, lift your feet from the mattress. Lower them. Where do you feel your muscles working?

Roll onto your side and curl up as much as you comfortably can. Now uncurl. Try this again on your other side.

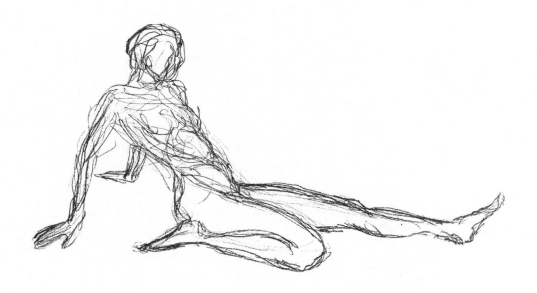

Sit up with your back against your headboard or the
wall. Bend your knees as much as you need to in order
to press the bottoms of your feet together. Keeping
your heels and toes touching, slide your feet as close to
you as you comfortably can. With your back supported
in bed, you will find it easier to explore various
stretches of this sort that require a strong back on
the open floor.

Lie on your back and imagine in vivid detail the first
enjoyable thing you want to do when you get up. Now
rise, stretch like a cat, and go do it.

How I begin

When I wake—usually quite early—I lie on my back in bed and do a bit of gentle stretching—spreading my legs, pointing my toes, extending my arms, rolling my shoulders. Then I wander barefoot out onto my little deck to see what the day looks like. Then I shower, giving my head a good massage as I wash my hair.

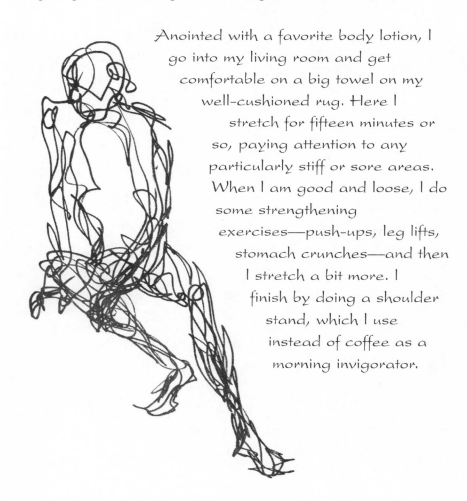

Anointed with a favorite body lotion, I go into my living room and get comfortable on a big towel on my well-cushioned rug. Here I stretch for fifteen minutes or so, paying attention to any particularly stiff or sore areas. When I am good and loose, I do some strengthening exercises—push-ups, leg lifts, stomach crunches—and then I stretch a bit more. I finish by doing a shoulder stand, which I use instead of coffee as a morning invigorator.

If I feel I have the time, I'll put on some music to match my mood and dance around for a while, stretching as I dance. If I get really involved and work up a good sweat, I'll take another quick shower before brewing a cup of tea and getting to work. I generally don't eat anything until midmorning.

I perform a similar routine before I go to bed, though I usually meditate afterward rather than dance. I find if I don't do some yoga before I go to bed, I may not sleep as well.

Though it took me several weeks to habituate myself to these routines, they make me feel so good, my body is now quite adamant that I stick to them whenever possible.

Relaxing into a stretch

The concept of relaxing while holding a stretch may be difficult to grasp until you've experienced it. Once you have, I think you'll find it extremely helpful to your practice.

Sit on your butt with your legs pointing straight out in front of you. Try to keep your back relatively straight. If this is difficult, sit with your back against a wall or sofa. Bending from the waist, reach forward as far as you can without straining, and gently grip your legs. When I begin this stretch, I usually can only comfortably reach as far as my knees.

Hold this initial stretch for several slow, deep breaths. Imagine the muscles in your legs relaxing. Sit back. Wait a moment. Choose a spot an inch or so beyond where you first stretched, and if it's fairly easy to do, reach to that spot, gripping your legs and holding the stretch. Remember not to strain. Your body is amazingly elastic, but there's no benefit in forcing it to stretch farther than it wants to.

Sit back, wait a moment, and now stretch forward as far as you can and grip your legs. Breathe deeply, and now—without releasing your grip—relax.

It seems to be our tendency to hold our entire self taut when any part of us is being fully stretched. By consciously deciding to relax while holding a stretch, you will probably find it easier to hold the stretch longer and extend it a little farther on your next try.

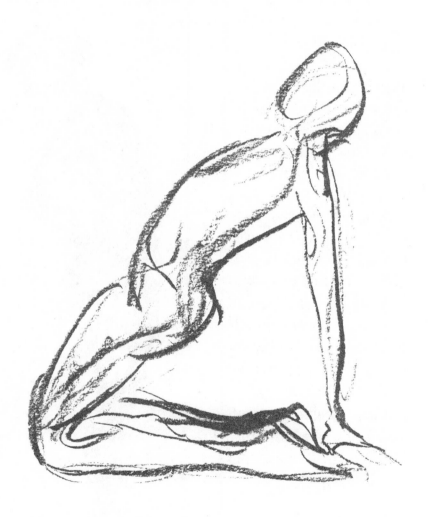

My locked back

I sometimes freeze in pain, or in fear of it, and I may stay frozen for several minutes before I remember: holding myself frozen usually makes the pain worse. Then I breathe deeply to relax, focusing my attention on what I perceive to be at the heart of my problem.

What's going on in my back? Does it feel like a nerve is being pinched? Is the pain like a hot poker jabbing me? Or is it a dull roar accompanied by vague numbness? The answers to these questions may determine whether ice or heat (or both) will help alleviate the pain. A word of caution: Ice should never be applied to a sore or distressed area for more than five minutes at a time. The reason for this is that your body will interpret too much cold as a trauma and react to protect itself.

Though it may be hard to imagine, temporary paralysis can sometimes be a blessing in disguise—an invaluable opportunity to review the choices I've made that brought me to this seemingly intractable condition. Being frozen, I cannot distract myself with other activities.

When I'm finally able to direct a calm, focused energy toward the distressed area—in this case, the muscles surrounding two vertebrae in my lower back—I sense small open spaces to either side of the bones involved. But when I stretch even slightly into one of these open spaces, fierce pain shoots up my back. So now what?

I relax into my immobility, remembering that every part of my body is connected to every other part by an amazingly efficient network of nerves and veins and arteries. I assure myself that if I work patiently with my body, and not against it, we will discover together what we must do.

As I contemplate my predicament, I interpret the jolt I experienced as a warning from my body to try something else. After a bit more rest, I decide on a less direct approach. I slowly raise my arms above my head until I feel the muscles in my upper back stretching. No pain. I raise them farther and then relax into a greater openness. Simultaneously, the blockage in my lower back lessens slightly.

Rather than force a stuck or severely painful place in your body to move, begin by stretching areas that are not painful. Loosening one area will have beneficial repercussions throughout your body.

Gradually work your way closer and closer to the problem zone, remembering not to strain. Rest frequently to let the impact of what you've done resonate fully.

It may take hours or days or weeks before a traumatized area is ready to be stretched or massaged directly. Be patient and trust in your body's healing powers. If you become discouraged, don't hesitate to consult an experienced physical therapist. I have had wonderful help over the years from massage therapists, acupuncturists, and chiropractors, though ultimately my healing was accomplished largely through my own efforts.

Breathing into places of pain

Sometimes I find it helpful to envision my pain as a physical entity that can be shrunk or dissolved or exorcised. At other times, it helps me to think of my pain as an expression of conflict—having no physical body of its own. This allows me to focus my attention on healing a place in my body rather than fighting a thing.

How ever we envision our pain, we can learn to direct our breath into places where pain locates itself. We can invite the energy comprising our pain to mount our breath and ride out on our exhalation.

Sometimes pain in one area goes away when another place is stretched or massaged. Pain will move from one site to another as we chase it with our changing postures and our intention to discover and expel it.

Stretching and breathing are partners in the exhumation and release of tension. Stretching expands the target for our breath.

Stretch gently around a tight place in your body. As you inhale, envision the molecules of air racing to the conflicted area to loosen and stimulate the painful tissues. As you exhale, imagine your breath carrying away your pain.

To enhance the practice of sending my breath to a particular place in my body, I will, if possible, touch that place with my fingers as I inhale. For whatever reason, touching the spot helps draw my breath there.

When you stretch before exercising, try sending your breath to the various parts of your body as you stretch them. Though Western medical doctors tell me that my breath cannot literally be traveling to places other than my lungs or stomach, visualizing my breath traveling throughout my body most definitely helps bring relief to troubled areas.

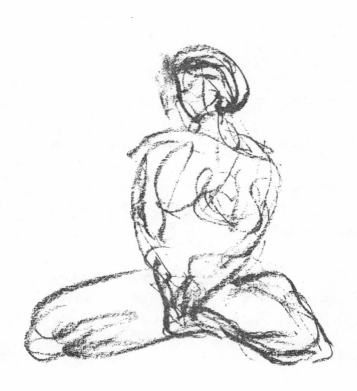

Helpful noise

I enjoy emptying myself—releasing tension—by humming or making a musical tone as I exhale.

Growling noises make good expellers of tension, too.

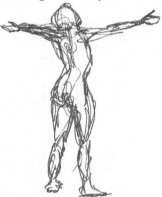

When I take a posture to the limits of my flexibility, I sometimes find myself holding my breath—a sure sign I'm not as relaxed as I might be. This is the reason yoga instructors constantly remind us to focus on breathing steadily and deeply as we stretch. To help myself remember, I have developed the habit of whispering, "Breathe," as I assume a posture.

Much to my delight, I have discovered that when I release my breath with a loud sound or musical tone, the exhalation is often more complete and salutary than if I try to discharge my breath silently.

I have also found that a good outcry often allows me to take a stretch farther than if I remain silent.

What are we eating?

Our personal relationship to food is an extremely important aspect of who we are and what we will become. After all, our bodies and brains are made from what we consume.

All food is energy suspended in precious water. Fruit is water saturated with tasty sugars. Meat is water dense with blood and fat and proteins. Fat is water laden with molecules of latent energy. Without some fat, we perish.

It seems that many people eat what their brains and taste buds tell them to eat and not what their bodies desire. Learning to distinguish between the two sources of inspiration is a key to creating healthful eating habits.

For instance, many vegetarians experience intense cravings for sugar. Eating cookies or ice cream may temporarily ease the craving, but it will quickly return because the body wants something else—usually protein, fat or a trace element their diet is lacking.

On the other end of the spectrum, heavy meat eaters are often prone to the use of stimulants—coffee, alcohol, sugar—because they feel the need for something to help them overcome the lethargy that often accompanies the consumption of large servings of meat. Their bodies, however, desire relief from so much fat and protein, and would much prefer vegetables and fruit to caffeine and sweets.

Here is an exercise that may help you become more conscious of your relationship to food.

Prepare a favorite meal. As you do so, be aware of the quality of the energy you bring to this task. Try slowing the process down. What makes this food so appealing to you? How old were you when it became a favorite? As you eat, pay attention to how you savor the taste of your favorite comestible.

After giving your body time for digestion, take a walk and imagine your food fueling your body, as if your organs comprise an exquisite engine. Do you feel satisfied, or are you still hungry for something?

I believe our bodies are supremely intelligent about what they need to function optimally. Sit comfortably and relax. Breathe deeply and relax further. Now ask your body what it needs in the way of sustenance. With practice, I think you will find that your body will tell you quite clearly what it needs.

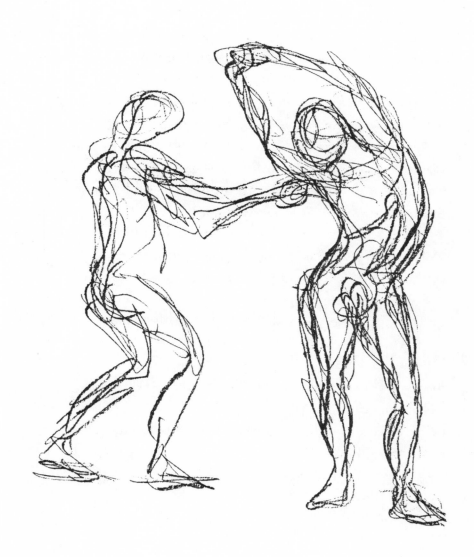

Water

The body, as you probably know, is comprised largely of water. All our lives, parents and teachers have told us to drink plenty of water. Unfortunately, many of us don't drink enough of the universal elixir.

Most people will say they drink water when they feel thirsty—when their throats are dry. But a dry throat is only one of the many ways our bodies call for water.

We often confuse hunger with thirst. The next time you're feeling peckish, drink a couple glasses of water and see if you still feel hungry.

When we suddenly feel warm or cold for no apparent reason, our body may be asking for water.

A feeling of lethargy may be the body calling for water.

Even minor aches and pains can sometimes be reduced or eliminated by drinking water.

Being properly hydrated will greatly enhance your physical flexibility, as well as your body's ability to communicate its more subtle needs.

Walking

Our bodies love to move. They were designed and perfected by nature to travel great distances with ease.

When we move, we ignite the dormant powers within us, and the body thrills to the prospect of fulfilling its potential.

Travel is the yoga of stretching yourself into new and refreshing geographies.

I try to do a bit of loosening up before I walk, but I'm often too eager to get going, so I stretch in transit— rolling my shoulders, swinging my arms, rotating my head, twisting my torso, and generally wiggling around.

I like to have a goal, a special halfway point in my walks. Sometimes I aim for a favorite bakery and the prospect of a magnificent muffin, but more often my destination is a favorite place to do some stretching or meditating, or both.

I used to live three miles from a deep, clear river, and my motivation for walking there on hot days was the bliss of diving into the cool waters and swimming slowly upstream.

Walking is a wonderful way to feel more grounded and to shake off minor depression and lethargy. Even a walk around the block will be much appreciated by your body.

And did you know that many of the greatest thinkers and artists throughout history have claimed that long walks were the catalysts for their most divine inspirations?

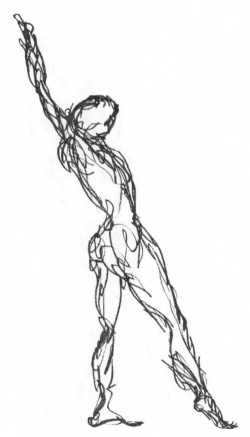

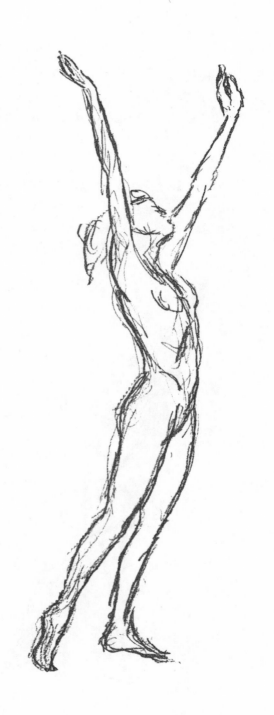

Honoring your body

Our bodies carry us through life, and we often take this heroic service for granted. Though we are not separate from our bodies, I advocate honoring the body as a divine animal, distinct from our personalities.

- ✎ I honor my body by giving it all the rest it needs.

- ✎ I honor my body by feeding it satisfying food and drink.

- ✎ I honor my body with warm baths.

- ✎ I honor my body by anointing it with soothing lotions.

- ✎ I care for my body as a loving mother cares for her baby.

- ✎ I honor my body by stretching and exercising.

- ✎ I honor my body with treatments from gifted healers.

- ✎ I honor my body by thanking it for helping me.

- ✎ I honor my body by dancing and singing.

- ✎ I honor my body by finding ways for it to play and commune with other bodies.

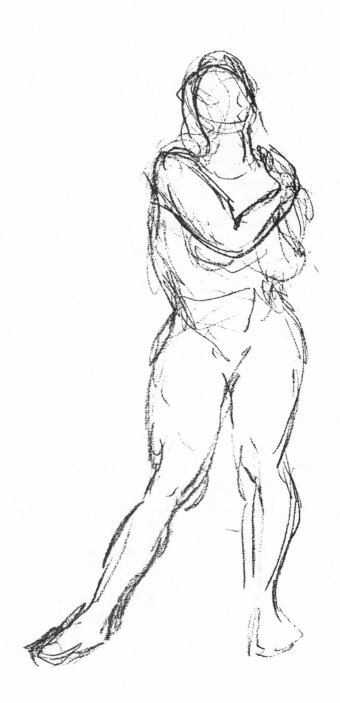

Self-massage

While giving myself massages, I often discover sore spots I would otherwise not have known about. Giving attention and touch to these less-obvious sites of pain can often help prevent greater discomfort later on.

Give yourself a head rub. Stimulating your scalp will free the upward flow of energies seeking release. You might do this in the shower while washing your hair. I like to start where my neck connects to my skull and slowly work my fingers up and over the top of my head to my forehead and temples, then down the side of my face to my jaw.

Sit comfortably and give yourself a foot massage. If you have trouble getting hold of your foot, this might be a worthy goal of your personal yoga.

Giving my hands a massage is one of my favorite ways to take a relaxing break from working at my desk.

Though it may not be as sensually satisfying as having someone else massage you, giving yourself a thorough massage—reaching as much of your body as you can—is a wonderful way to invigorate yourself while stretching and strengthening your arms and hands.

Balancing

As I suggested at the beginning of this book, we sit or stand or move the way we do for comfort and balance. This is a natural response to directives from our body, but if these postures favor one side or one limb, and we don't practice the opposite or balancing postures, imbalance will become difficult to amend.

If we are dedicated to attending a yoga class, and we do as our instructor demonstrates, our bodies will inform us of many things—weakness, stiffness, imbalance. But there is nothing so revealing as the poses we choose constantly in our daily lives. And there is nothing so convenient as reacting yogically—on the spot—to what we discover.

Though pain and tension are certainly symptoms of physical imbalance, our emotional and intellectual activities may also require adjustments before we can feel fully balanced. Taking time to do yoga is a way to begin balancing yourself.

Sit on the floor with your legs pointing straight in front of you. You may wish to sit against a wall if it's more comfortable for you. Keeping your back straight, look at your knees and the heels of your feet. Are they aligned with each other? If not, shift your legs so they are. Hold. How does it feel when your legs are symmetrically aligned?

Stand comfortably in front of a mirror. Is one shoulder higher than the other? If so, bring your shoulders into symmetrical alignment. Hold. How does that feel?

I like to think we have two legs, two arms, two hands, two knees, two feet, and two shoulders to assist us in balancing ourselves. If you feel grossly out of balance with yourself, and no amount of stretching seems to help, you may need a good rest. Take a day off and relax. If that doesn't help, you may wish to visit a good body worker for a tune-up.

While physically balancing yourself, try meditating on actions you might take to balance other areas of your life. This may involve beginning or complet- ing a task, calling someone you want to make contact with, taking more time to meditate, or remem- bering to take your vitamins.

Our bodies invariably reflect our emotional lives. When we're happy, our bodies usually feel terrific. If we're procrastinating, we tend to feel stiff or tired. If we're afraid to do something, or to make a change we know would be good for us, we tend to feel anxious and hold ourselves stiffly, which leads to soreness and may interfere with our sleep. When we are preoccupied and not fully present, we are more prone to accidents because we are unaware of warnings from our bodies.

Taking just a few minutes each day to sit or stand in a balanced posture can often help bring an unconscious emotional imbalance to our attention. Then, using our good intentions, we can move to remedy it.

Sitting in a comfy chair

When I ask a person, "How are you sitting?" they almost always make some sort of physical shift. Sometimes they sit up straighter. Sometimes they pull their shoulders back. Sometimes they cross or uncross their legs. You may have made a shift when you read the question. But how were you sitting before the question entered your consciousness?

Sit in your favorite chair. Get comfortable. Hold this pose until it stops feeling good. Try to identify where in your body your discomfort is centered before you change position. How does your new pose ameliorate your discomfort? You are discovering the yoga you have been practicing all your life. You are assuming postures from which you may be able to do some highly beneficial stretching.

A stable chair with arms is wonderful for certain stretches. Sitting with uncrossed legs, feet on the floor, place your hands palms down on the arms of your chair and push against the arms to help flatten your back against the back of the chair. Use this pressure against the arms to hold your back flat. Release and repeat.

From the same position, put both hands on the right arm of the chair and pull against the arm to twist your torso to the right. Relax. Keeping your hands on the right arm of the chair, twist to the left. Now put both hands on the left arm of the chair to enhance your twisting to the left, and then after relaxing, twist to the right.

I have a high-backed armchair I like to kneel on, facing the back of the chair. I use the sides and top of the chair to help me hold sideways stretches, and to balance me while I arch my back.

On this same high-backed armchair, I will lie on my back with my butt touching the bottom of the chair back, my legs extended up the back of the chair, my head hanging over the edge of the chair. This is a great way to elevate my legs and stretch my neck.

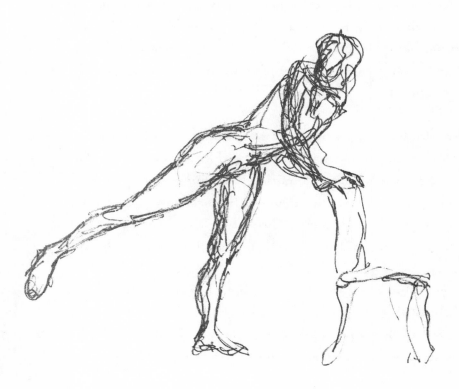

Be sure to approach all your new postures carefully and slowly. A new posture will often reveal long-unstretched and untested parts of your body. Strive for balance and comfort, and when completing a chair pose, exit slowly so you don't fall.

One of my favorite positions is to sit facing forward in a big armchair, or as it is known in my house, a solo sofa. I like to bring my feet up on the seat so my heels touch my butt. Sometimes I hug my knees, sometimes I don't. I love this posture because it makes me feel young and mischievous. I used to sit like this when I was younger and more mischievous than I am now.

Staying in this posture, I flatten my back against the back of the chair. Then I place my hands behind my head and press my elbows back to help open my chest.

After I stretch in various directions from this posture for ten or fifteen minutes, my body is usually ready to sit quietly for a spell of meditation.

Tools

Chairs aren't the only handy devices for enhancing our stretching and meditating. Glance through a yoga magazine or yoga catalogue and you will see advertisements for various sizes and shapes of pillows and chunks of foam, balls, slant boards, curved-backed tables, inversion devices, and other goodies to assist you in bending and stretching.

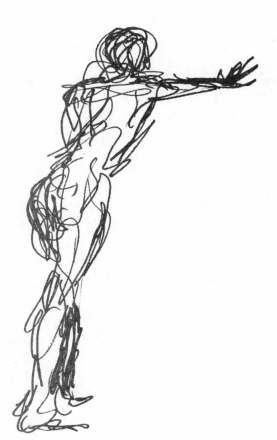

However, most of the things I use to help me stretch are already in my possession, or I find them as I make my way through the world.

I use a basketball for all sorts of stretches. The ball helps me maintain my balance and gives me something perfectly round and resilient to push against. Holding a ball aloft encourages me to stretch farther than when I don't hold a ball.

I sometimes use a sturdy oak staff, five feet long, for centering and balancing postures. I find that using a staff or a pole, either for support or held in both hands as I stretch and twist, adds a satisfying, ritualistic feel to my practice.

When I'm waiting for a train, I like to squat and flatten my back against a wall. Even a few minutes of squatting is a great relief after walking or standing all day.

I use doorknobs for balance when I squat and twist.

I like to hang from a bar to decompress my spine.

Hanging my head off the end of a bench or bed helps open my neck and shoulders.

Placing my hands on both sides of a doorway and leaning through the opening makes for a satisfying, chest-opening stretch.

The poles of bus stop signs make good stretching posts. I grasp the pole, one hand above the other, place my feet side by side at the base of the pole, and bend at the waist, remembering to keep my back straight. With each subsequent stretch, I lower my hands a little farther down the pole until I reach a comfortable limit to my flexibility.

Using walls and pillows and balls and poles in my yoga adds an element of creative play, which makes the process much more interesting and fun.

Gravity

An important goal of yoga is to get our feet above our heads. We all know how good it feels to put our feet up after a day of upright toil, but it's not only our lower appendages that benefit from this altitude shift. Our entire body rejoices when we reverse our usual circulation scenario.

Popular asanas for switching the positions of head and feet are the shoulder stand and the head stand. For many people, though, these are advanced positions. If you wish to try these postures, make sure your neck and back are loose and warm, and please consider having a friend assist you at first. You may also wish to enlist the aid of a wall.

A less difficult way to elevate your legs is to lie on your back on the floor with your feet up on the seat of a chair.

I once severely sprained my left foot, causing it to swell to twice the size of my right foot. To alleviate my discomfort, I would elevate my feet high above my head, and I could watch the swollen foot shrink to the size of my other foot.

Inverting the body, however you safely accomplish this, will enhance the circulation in your lungs and increase the supply of oxygenated blood to your brain. I find this cerebral infusion extremely helpful to my mental functioning.

Coils

Sometimes I envision my body as an assemblage of springs which tend to coil tightly unless I regularly pull them apart.

Reach your arms toward the ceiling. Stretch your fingers. What are your shoulders saying? Your back? The base of your spine? Your buttocks? Your legs? All your parts are speaking. Calm yourself and listen carefully.

Press the fingers of your right hand against the fingers of your left. Do you feel the little coils separating? What is the sensation you feel in the spaces you've created?

Stand comfortably. Close your eyes. Envision the coiled springs that comprise your whole body. When you have a clear image of these springs, imagine there is a light as bright as the sun in the center of your chest. Now imagine this light flowing through your body and warming the coils.

When I feel internally warm, my stretching is always more enjoyable and effective. If you're feeling particularly stiff and cold, you might wish to take a warm bath or shower before you begin your stretching.

Coiling and uncoiling

In a bath, in bed, anywhere—imagine your entire body is a single coil, one spring to be wound or unwound. Note that "wound" and "wound" are spelled identically, yet one means a tightening, the other means an injury—aspects of the same phenomenon. When a part of us is wounded, it coils tightly to defend itself.

Where are you the tightest? Where are you most flexible? Where do you feel most uncomfortable about being touched?

Tighten the entire coil that comprises your being. Tighten every atom. Coil yourself and now

uncoil!

Do this again and again until you grow warmer.

I find it wonderfully grounding to experience my body as a single entity, as well as a collection of parts.

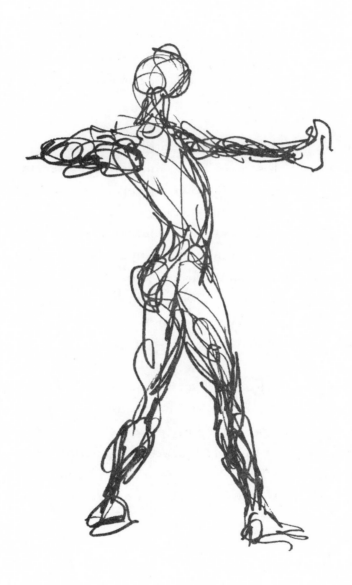

Grounding

When we are grounded we feel calm and fully connected to the earth and to ourselves. It is a simple concept, yet for many people becoming grounded is difficult.

Standing barefoot on the ground, on a rug, or on the floor helps ground us. Imagine that you can send energy from your body down through your feet into the earth. Now imagine the reverse—energy flowing up through your feet from the earth. Face toward the west and inhale deeply, releasing your breath with a low, steady hum. Now face north. Inhale, and release your breath with a hum. Now face east and repeat the process, and now south to complete the cycle.

Another way I ground myself is to kneel and arch my back, placing my hands on the ground behind me. Holding this pose, I close my eyes, relax, and then stretch farther, staying focused on an image of a favorite place in the wilderness. When I come out of this posture, I almost always feel grounded and grateful.

There are many healers who believe that the source of much of our physical and emotional discomfort is the direct result of a lack of connection to the earth itself.

For some people, taking a walk, even a short one, can
be wonderfully grounding.

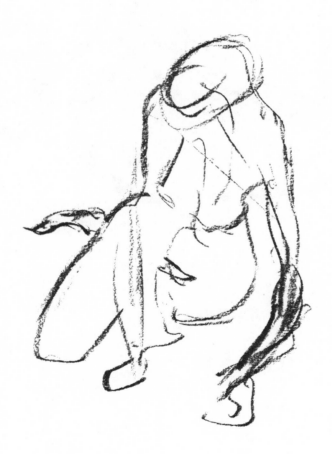

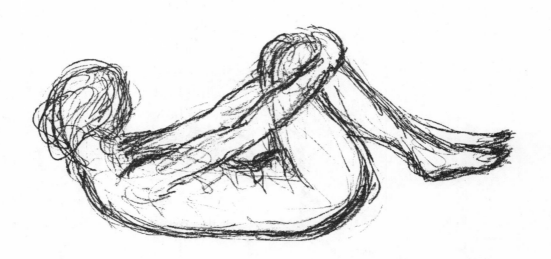

Centering

When I was learning how to use a potter's wheel, the first thing to master was the centering of a ball of clay from which everything would be made. What did this entail?

First, I had to place the ball of clay in the center of the wheel. Second, I had to physically align myself directly and symmetrically above the ball of clay. Third, I had to kick the treading stone in a confident and rhythmically steady way. Fourth, I had to apply even pressure to the clay with both my hands. Finally, and most importantly, I had to be centered in myself.

How did I feel when I was finally able to center the ball of clay? I felt calm, free of doubt, fully present, and in absolute harmony with all parts of the process, and therefore not separate from it.

Sit comfortably, breathing slowly and deeply. Close your eyes and imagine that you live in your brain. Now intentionally make a journey out of your head and down to your heart. Imagine that in your heart you dissolve into tiny pieces carried by your blood to every cell in your body. You enliven your cells, and they enliven you, and you return to your heart where you coalesce into your whole self again.

Here. In your heart. Centered.

Origins

I believe that much of my early physical stiffening was caused by extreme emotional distress. Our bodies act spontaneously to protect us. If our hearts are broken, our shoulders will close around our chests and we will hold ourselves in tense anticipation of further trauma: a surefire prescription for pain and ill health.

I reached my most expansive physical and emotional state at the age of ten. I was strong, limber, bright, self-confident, and madly in love with life. I was four feet six inches tall. I weighed seventy-four pounds and could scamper effortlessly to the tops of the tallest trees.

It was at this point in my development that my relatively carefree childhood came swiftly to a close. Following a series of traumatic injuries—a fall from a tree onto my back, having my sternum crushed under the knee of a bully, fracturing my heel in a neighborhood track meet—I began the difficult journey into adulthood with its requisite confusion and unavoidable sorrows.

At twelve I was still an ambitious athlete, though my rigidity was considerable by then. I played center field on our school baseball team, halfback on our football team, and I held the school record for pull-ups and the pole climb.

At thirteen, I could high-jump nearly six feet. I did so awkwardly, but I could do it.

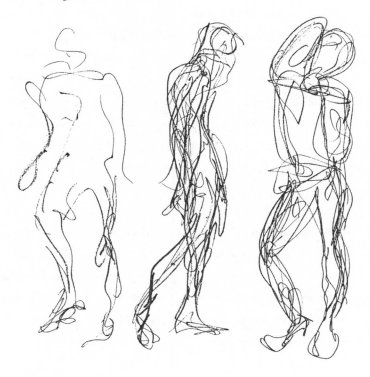

Fourteen. High school. I rode my bicycle for hours every day, running away to nowhere. School felt like prison to me, and I was in constant conflict with my parents. They wanted me to study more and show an interest in science and math, while I wanted to play basketball and be an actor. It was at this time that I began to experience subtle aches and pains when I woke in the morning.

Fifteen. I went on a backpack trip with two friends in the hot, dry mountains behind Big Sur. I woke each morning almost too stiff to move, but I'd be free of pain after I took three aspirin and walked around for a while.

Then came the tackle football game where my stiffening joints took one too many punishing blows and my body became inflamed where the fusing was most advanced—in my lower back and hips.

Though I may never know how much of my physical disability was the result of psychological stress, I share the belief of many healers that our emotional state has an enormous impact on our physical well-being. I think it is highly worthwhile to investigate through meditation, and perhaps with the help of a therapist, the psychological underpinnings of our physical histories.

Releasing

Injuries, insults, rejection, shame, fear. We hold them in
our muscles, our nerves, our cells, our blood, our bones,
our lungs, our hearts. Our imagination is a tool for see-
ing these things as entities within us, affixed to places
of pain. We may gather these entities on our breath
and release them. We may soothe the ache of ensuing
emptiness with new breath.

Stretch to open a place of pain.
Now imagine your breath carrying
light inside you, a warm light
that engages your pain and
softens it. Now exhale
your pain with a shout.

I've learned over the years that much
of my pain resides in
unreleased rage. To help me
release this pent-up fury, I have
modified a process taught to me
by a therapist. I will gather
several cardboard boxes and
kneel on a pillow before
them. I take a sturdy stick,
two feet long, and grasp
one end of it with both
hands. Shouting as I strike,
I demolish the boxes. This

is my chance to symbolically fight back against all the abuse—physical and verbal—I was unable to defend myself against at the time of the original assaults because I was too small or hurt or afraid. I strike and shout and verbalize my anger until I feel relieved. Then I strike and shout some more. I am usually free of pain after a good session of releasing rage.

If you try smashing cardboard boxes or bashing old telephone books, give it all you've got. Afterward, stretch your arms, legs, and back, and then take a warm bath. You may be a bit sore the next day, but it's worth it.

Mental yoga

The brain is a fabulous instrument, generating tens of thousands of thoughts each day. It has been discovered, however, that nearly all our thoughts are the same ones we had yesterday. We are truly creatures of habit. One might surmise that repetitive mental patterns freeze our personalities in the same way that redundant physical choices freeze our bodies.

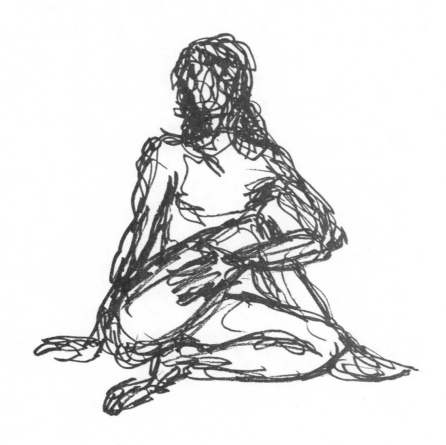

Sometimes I'll get stuck in my writing and I'll try switching the pen to my left hand. Though it is
physically more difficult for me, it is quite stimulating to
my thought process—further proof of the profound link
between our brains and our bodies.

In yoga, after we twist in one direction, we try to twist
in the other direction to balance our musculature. I like
to practice this mentally, too. When I find myself fixed
on a certain point of view, I try to elucidate, without
judgment, its opposite. Doing so may not change my
mind, but it certainly stretches me, quite often to good
effect.

The heroic being

A dear friend confessed, "If I don't force my body to exert itself, I will sit inert, staring into space or at the tube, eating mindlessly until I turn into a pain-ridden slug."

"But what if," I mused in response, "we see our bodies as heroic beings, with heroic habits. What if every night before sleeping, we imagine our bodies to be the powerful guardians of our souls. And through these bodies, with the help of our ingenious brains, we fulfill our souls' desires."

"How do you define 'soul'?" my friend asked, closing his eyes to give himself over to the idea.

"I define soul as those parts of us transcendent of our physical bodies, reflected in our personalities and our imaginations and our desires."

"And what exactly are heroic habits?" he asked, opening his eyes and smiling. "Doing fifty sit-ups every day?"

"Or rising each morning and doing twenty minutes of yoga, eating well, walking or riding our bicycles to do our errands, taking samba lessons."

"And how would these habits help fulfill my soul's desire?"

"Well, that would depend on what your soul desired."

"And how, pray tell, does one determine that?"

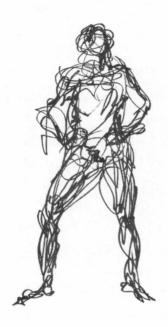

"Well, you might meditate on the question, What do I really want to do? Not what do I want? or what do I want to be? But what do I want to do? Not what do I think I *should* do, but what do I want to do?"

"And what if I come up with eating mindlessly while watching the tube?"

"Then do it. Though after a few days of heroic habits, I'll bet you come up with something else."

Intentional Pain

My friend Vance was pondering the idea of pain as part of his body's language. Suddenly, he looked up with a light in his eyes and said, "Don't forget to mention intentional pain. When your body wants to ache tomorrow as proof you worked it well today."

"Should it be a painful aching?"

"Maybe pain isn't quite the right word," he continued. "I mean that feeling of having exercised hard enough—a somewhat heavy tautness—that makes me want to stretch to keep from tightening up."

Whatever we choose to call those sensations our bodies experience in the aftermath of rigorous exercise—pain or soreness or aching or heaviness or muscular fatigue—fitness experts agree that giving our bodies a strenuous workout two or three times a week (stretching thoroughly before and after) dramatically increases our chances of remaining free of debilitating pain or stiffness.

If you are not in the habit of exercising strenuously but wish to begin doing so, be careful not to push yourself too hard for too long at first. Walking briskly for fifteen minutes is a much saner way to begin pushing your body than to suddenly try to run a mile or two.

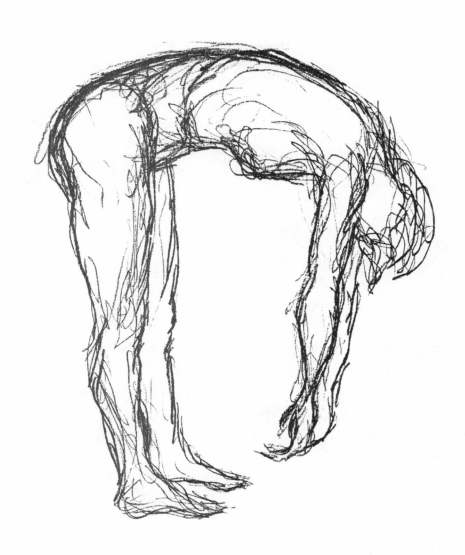

Whatever kind of exercise you choose, be sure to check in with your body every few minutes to see how it's doing. This doesn't mean you need to stop doing what you're doing. Merely slow down a bit so you can better sense how your body is feeling.

I also recommend what I call preemptive physical evaluations. If a friend invites you to go on a ten-mile hike and you're unsure whether you're capable of such an adventure—but you might be—relax for a few minutes and pose the question to your body. Imagine yourself doing what you've been invited to do. If grave doubts arise, see if there aren't ways to modify the adventure to make it less daunting, but still a good challenge.

The big refill

Once, I was stretching by the fire, taking a posture farther than I'd ever dared take it before. I could feel something in my spine resisting the pressure of my bending. At first, I believed the resistance to be a kind of pain. I grimaced in reaction to the sensation, but then I realized the resistance was not particularly painful. It was my anticipation of pain that caused me to grimace. I was afraid. So I relaxed and listened to my body.

"Go on," it said. "You won't hurt yourself."

I resumed the posture, opening myself until the sensation of blockage seemed to fill my entire back. I took a deep breath and opened farther, and something gave way with an audible pop. I was very warm by then, sweating profusely. I lay on my back and breathed deeply into the place where the blockage had been centered. There seemed to be a huge space there now, hungry to be filled with breath and light.

An hour later, a friend came by, gave me a hug, and said, "Am I crazy, or are you taller?"

"Yes," I replied. "Absolutely."

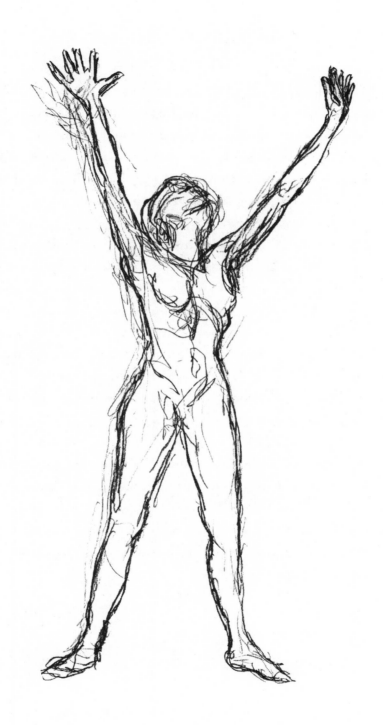

Walking in the waves

Every now and then I'll take the bus to the beach. The warm sand makes a wonderful yoga studio. I like to lie on my back, with my feet slightly uphill if possible, and slowly wiggle my back and butt to create a comfortable indentation in which to do my stretching. The sand is so accommodating—yielding, yet supportive.

I often meet other people at the beach doing yoga or giving themselves beach-assisted back adjustments. Some prefer to do their work on a big towel or blanket; others enjoy direct contact with the sand.

Once I'm comfortable and loose, I like to go walking along the sand where the waves rush up to spend the last of the energy they've carried over the ocean for hundreds of miles.

What I call my sideways muscles get nicely exercised as I walk and run through the shallows, the inrushing and outrushing tide pulling at my ankles and calves and knees. And along with the exercise, I get to gawk at the miraculous ocean and commune with my fellow water worshippers.

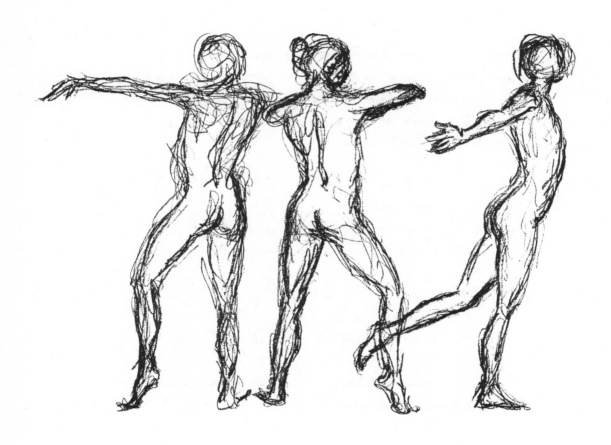

Water yoga

If you are fortunate to have access to a swimming pool, you'll be able to do all sorts of slow and graceful movements with your body that you'd never be able to do out of water.

Most adults think of swimming pools as places to swim laps, but when it comes to water yoga, I defer to my younger teachers. What do most children spontaneously choose to do when given a swimming pool to play in?

- They spend most of their time having fun in the shallow end.

- They practice holding their breath underwater.

- They try to stand on their hands.

- They exhale completely and sink to the bottom.

- They swoop through the water, imagining they are flying.

- They float on their backs and stare up at the sky.

- They try to walk and run through the water.

✍ They spin around in circles.

✍ They leap and dive.

✍ They shout for joy.

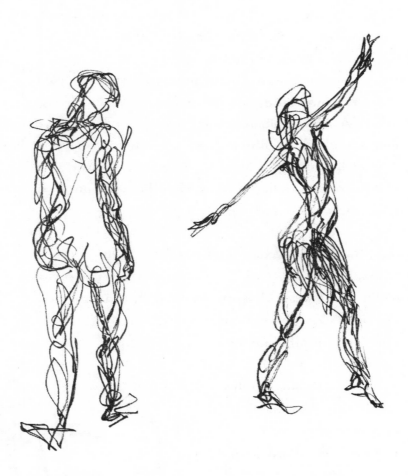

Young teachers

I spent a most instructive year as a teacher's aide in a day-care center for children ages two to five years old. I was often the sole caretaker of dozens of these delightful beings, and so to maximize my effectiveness, I devised various methods of crowd control.

Stretching Time was one of the most popular group activities I instituted, second only to Running from the Tickle Monster (me). During Stretching Time, I would invite the children to mimic my movements and postures. Most of the children were so limber compared to me, their greatest challenge was to sufficiently understate my asanas.

Then I would let each of them take a turn as the "teacher," and we would all imitate whatever pose or stretch our leader demonstrated. What astonishing yoga masters these children were! What inspiring flexibility we are born to.

To this day, I love doing yoga with children. For their part, they seem to delight in this kind of play with a big person.

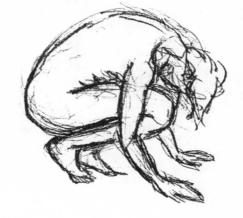

Dance yoga

Imagine that music contains wordless instructions for how to move and loosen your body so that your stiffness will lessen and eventually disappear.

Remember that we are all evolved from people who spent a good deal of their free time singing and dancing.

Making sounds came before language.

The emotion of sound needs no literal translation.

Allow yourself to sing your feelings by making whatever noises you wish to make. How does your body want to move when you make certain sounds? Let your sound making inspire your body movements.

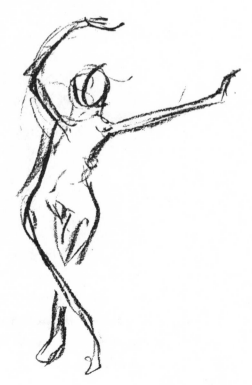

For my kind of stiffness, nothing loosens me so profoundly as a good, long, wiggling dance.

Yoga parties

Invite friends over for a group stretching session. Tell everybody to wear loose, comfortable clothes, and to bring their favorite mats and pillows.

Gather in the most spacious room and encourage everyone to sprawl and loll comfortably for a while. When everyone feels relaxed and present, share postures you've each discovered, and describe how they make you feel.

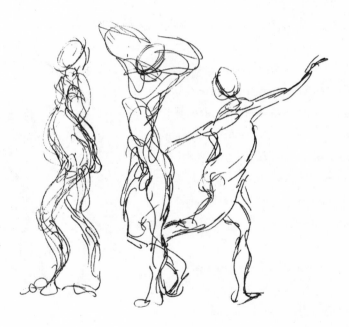

No one will be able to do anyone else's posture exactly, but everyone can do his or her personal version of the original.

Take turns sharing these postures and assisting each other until everyone feels warmer. Now hum and sing together, harmonizing wordlessly, releasing energy together through joyful noise.

Share a simple meal and discuss your latest discoveries about your bodies.

After the food has settled, put on some rhythmic music and let the dancing begin.

Lily's posture

Here is a posture I learned at a yoga party. Please read this description slowly. It sounds more complicated than it is.

Sitting on her butt on the floor, her legs facing forward, Lily crooks her right knee and places her right foot across her left thigh. Holding her right foot with her left hand, and keeping her back straight, she leans forward and tries to touch her left foot with her right hand. She holds this stretch for a minute or so before returning to a relaxed sitting position.

Then she switches legs, crooking her left knee and placing her left foot across her right thigh. Holding her left foot with her right hand, she leans forward and tries to touch her right foot with her left hand. Alternating legs, and never straining, she is eventually able to grasp the extended foot.

Lily explained how she discovered the posture. "I was having terrible back pain. After much experimentation, I discovered that this was a way I could sit and not be in too much pain. I would do this for a long time every day, and after a few weeks, my pelvis, back and arms felt much stronger and more flexible, and I felt much less pain. I do it for ten minutes a day now. Maintenance."

Circle

Talking in a circle is a yoga of community. Make a circle with two or more people, and declare it safe and sacred.

Even if you already know each other, go around the circle and briefly introduce yourselves. Now go around the circle sharing anything you feel like sharing. Memories. Stories. New thoughts. Songs. Questions. Sounds.

When I participate in a sharing circle, I remind myself that I can give a gift to my friends by honoring their words as I hope they will honor mine.

Each of us has a practice of speech and a practice of listening. It is a wonderful challenge to bring these complementary processes into balance with each other.

Listening

A good way to begin a conversation is to ask a question, and then listen openly and patiently to the answer.

The yoga of conversation is the union of minds and spirits through the messages we convey with words.

To listen as much as I talk is a great challenge for me.

All of us want to be recognized, accepted, listened to, and loved. It's the least we can do for each other.

I am often so eager to speak, I don't hear everything the other person wishes to communicate. Or I respond to what they begin to say without allowing them to finish their thought. I remind myself that allowing a bit of silence before responding can help establish a rhythm of conversation in which I more fully appreciate what each person has to say.

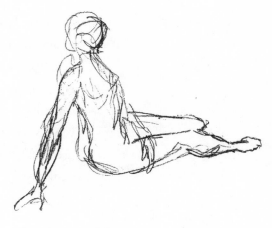

Yoga for two

Having chosen a willing and trusty compadre, stand facing each other and loosen up by mimicking each other's movements and facial expressions. Within moments, you will be mimicking each other's mimicry.

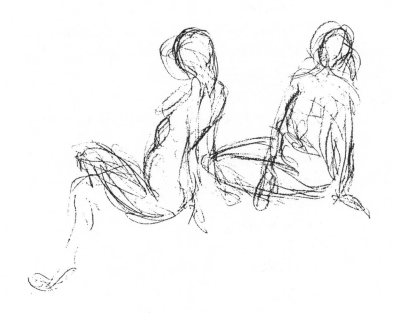

Standing a foot or so apart, raise your hands to the level of your faces, palms facing forward, and press your fingers against your partner's fingers. Exert enough pressure to create a comfortable balance between you. Now lean forward until your foreheads touch. Remember to breathe slowly and deeply. After you've held this pose for a time, count to three and gracefully push away from each other.

Stand back-to-back, butt to butt, and join hands. From this position, stretch together, seeking balance. Take turns allowing one of you to gently bend or pull the other.

As you try various stretches together, describe where you experience pain or stiffness.

Yoga for two gives us a wonderful opportunity to merge our intentions and move beyond barriers we've discovered in our aloneness.

A good hug is a crucial posture for all of us to explore.

More yoga for two

Yoga for two bodies is also yoga for two spirits.

Lie side by side on your backs, barely touching each other. Breathe deeply and open yourself to your partner's energy. Talk quietly about how your bodies are feeling and what postures you'd like to try together.

Demonstrate a favorite posture for your friend and ask for assistance in extending the stretch. For instance, when I lie on my stomach, reaching my arms straight behind me, I want to expand my ability to lift my head

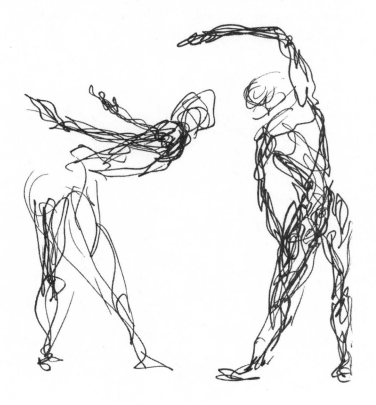

and arch my back. My partner, assuming her own comfortable position, can take hold of my hands and pull gently, helping me lift and stretch much farther than I can on my own.

I also like to have help when I'm standing on one leg, lifting and extending the other leg behind me. I like my partner to lift my extended leg up so I can hold the pose longer and extend the stretch.

Partnering is great for all kinds of postures involving balance and holding a pose for an extended period of time. While assisting someone, remember never to strain or hold your body in an uncomfortable position. The stances you take when helping your partner should also be beneficial to you.

Sex and yoga

A great combination

Sensual exploration of each other
with complete mutual trust

Sharing secrets of what feels good where

Creating mutually satisfying postures

Harmonizing words and sounds with pleasing actions

Fully present

Free

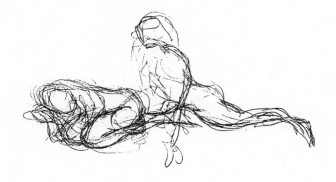

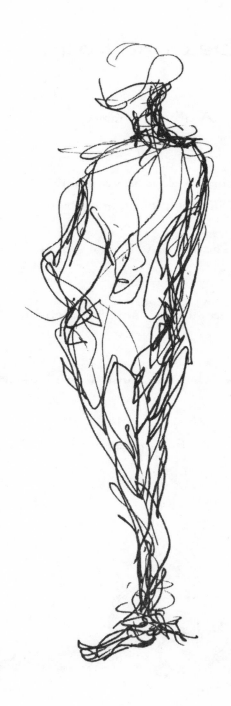

The practice of being alone

Being alone is a communion between your body, which has weight and form, and your personality, which is weightless and manifests as sound and gesture, thoughts and feelings.

Feel your pulse by placing the palm of your left hand against your throat. Press gently with your thumb. This is the sensation of your heart irrigating your body with blood—the rich red water of life. Your veins and arteries are the tributaries of great rivers of blood that spring from all you consume, all you feel, all you believe.

How do you wish to move through life?

How do you want others to receive you?

Stand comfortably and look out a window. Open yourself to change. Wait until you receive a signal to move. This signal may come from your body, or it may come in the form of a new thought. Or perhaps something will move through your field of vision. Change position. Take a deep breath and exhale fully.

It's good to be alone.

Public yoga

A friend once told me that after several failed relationships, she finally realized that she would never be capable of having a successful relationship with another person until she first developed a successful relationship with herself. Certainly one of the benefits of learning to accept and enjoy my aloneness has been the greater ease and confidence I feel about going out into the world. My relationship to the greater human community has definitely been enhanced by my improved relationship with myself.

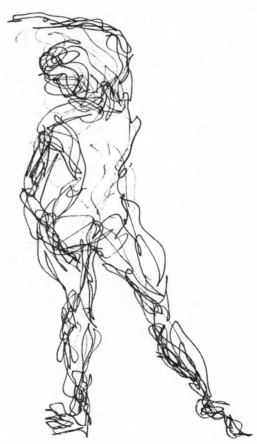

I never used to stretch in public, but over time my desire to be free of pain has overcome my self-consciousness. Now I do my yoga everywhere— while I'm waiting for a train, in the grocery store, on a walk around the block. Sometimes a person will see me stretching, and he or she will reflexively stretch, too. Perhaps stretching, like yawning, is contagious.

Yoga relieves me, and when I'm relieved I feel better, and when I feel better I have more energy to share, which makes me a better friend, a better stranger.

One morning, while I was using the pole of a bus-stop sign to help me stretch, a man waiting for the bus asked me if I knew anything he could do for his stiff neck. With his permission, I gave him a gentle neck and shoulder massage, after which I showed him how, by holding his head with both hands, he could carefully roll his head to loosen his neck. His smile of relief was a great beginning to my day.

Advanced positions

I may never be able to assume many of the more advanced yoga postures. Indeed, I have hurt myself trying to assume some of them. This, one might argue, is the problem with assumptions. But seriously, it is essential to the maintenance of my personal yoga to remind myself, as often as necessary, that I am not Swami Anybody Else, and that as of this writing I cannot bend backwards and rest my forehead on the bottom of my feet.

To practice my personal yoga, I must start where I am and proceed from there.

What I can assume are advanced versions of my own postures—beautiful and unique versions that are testaments to my progress.

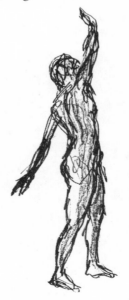

Alone again

Take a little time to meditate on the purpose of your yoga. Others can guide you by demonstrating physical patterns that may help you, but only you can respond to the subtle and intimate needs of your body.

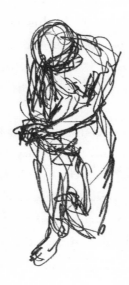

Stand quietly and relax. As you inhale, imagine the air falling like a waterfall through your body, cleansing you. Now imagine this air rising through you, rushing to your head, swirling around in your skull, refreshing your brain and face and eyes before you exhale.

Being alone has nothing to do with loneliness. Indeed, learning to love my aloneness has been the cure for my loneliness—for we are never alone, connected as we are to everything else.

The home stretch

What am I holding onto that no longer serves me? An idea? A feeling? A memory? A way of holding my body?

Stand comfortably, breathing slowly and deeply. Allow a feeling to announce itself. Is this feeling coming from a particular place in your body? Move your arms and neck and shoulders and back and feet. Where do you feel a catch or stiffness? Answer the loudest call.

Sometimes our bodies wish to move, to be in open air, to see what happens as we journey into the unknown. Some of our pain may reside in our fear of change. Is there something you'd really like to do but can't quite work up the energy or courage to begin? Is there some small step you could take in the direction of fulfilling your desire?

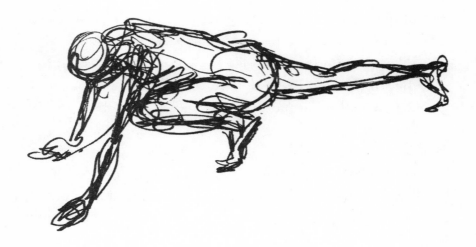

What is it about change that frightens us? Perhaps we can we begin to transform this fear into curiosity.

However you find yourself today, stretch open and breathe. Imagine yourself filling with the energy for action. Now envision yourself—the person you love—moving fearlessly through life.

Healers

There are times in our lives when we decide to seek help from others in order to heal more rapidly, more fully. Having had few positive experiences with medical doctors, I tend to seek care from alternative health-care providers whenever possible. Within the categories of body workers, chiropractors, acupuncturists and psychotherapists, there are myriad variations and combinations of techniques and healing philosophies. Finding and making effective use of a skillful healer is well worth your effort. Here are a few tips that may prove helpful.

- Ask friends for recommendations. If someone you trust believes they have been helped by a healer, give that person a try. Sometimes a friend may recommend a particular kind of treatment, and a search through the phone book may reveal a nearby practitioner of that school of healing.

- When you meet your healer, describe your pain or problem as thoroughly as you can. Bring along a written chronology of events pertaining to your difficulty, and be sure to describe your lifestyle and habits. Skillful healers are almost always good listeners and explainers. If you don't feel a healer is listening to you, he or she may not be worth your time and money.

≈ Trust your intuition and the responses of your body. Do you feel safe in this healer's care? How does your body feel when this person touches you? How does your body feel the next day? If after a treatment or two, you experience no positive change, you may wish to seek another healer.

≈ Following a visit to your healer, try not to get in a car right away. Take a walk or sit quietly, allowing your body to integrate more fully the healing it has received.

≈ Work with your healer. Keep them updated on how you and your body are doing. It is extremely important that you remain the master of your own care. If you feel you are not making progress, ask questions, seek other solutions, and leave any situation you feel is counter-productive.

≈ All skillful healers agree that a most important factor in healing is the level of faith a client has in his or her practitioner. Do you feel your healer respects you and cares about you? Do you feel you can trust them with the intimate details of your life? If not, why not? True healing is an intimate act.

≈ Integrate your own healing practices—your yoga— with the healing treatments you receive. Remember: You are working with yourself twenty-four hours a day. You are your primary caregiver.

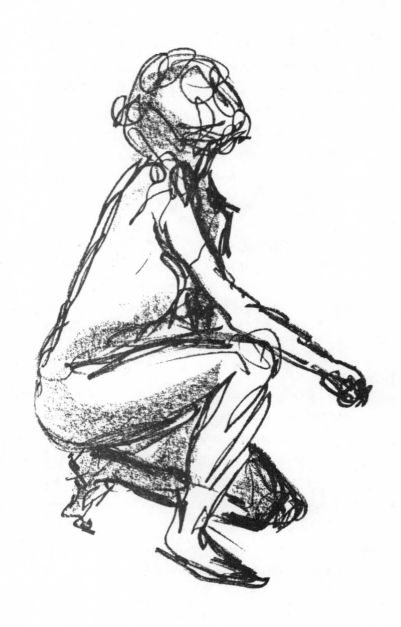

Gratitude

thank you for the breath of life

thank you for those who gave us life

thank you for our faithful bodies

thank you for our loving friends

thank you for our generous hearts
and our creative minds

thank you for warm and tender memories

thank you for this sacred earth

thank you for the divine nature of existence

thank you for every precious moment

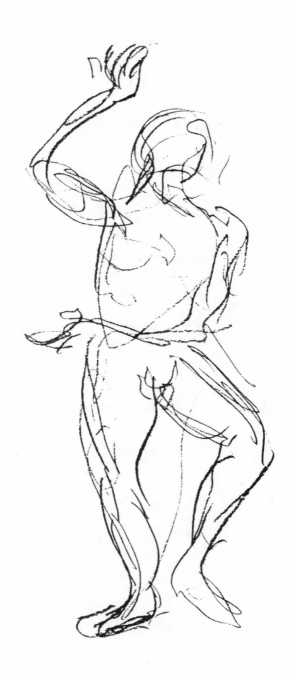

Blessings

Many dear friends contributed to the critical mass of ideas and experiences that prompted me to write this book.

I would especially like to thank Vance Lawry for his evocative works of art, Robin DeVol for her inspiring massage, Linda Danziger for her great heart, and Mindy Toomay for her devotion and support.

My editor, Lyssa Keusch, was a marvelous collaborator, as was my agent, Laurie Fox.

David Jouris, John Grimes, Robin Chin, Tad Toomay, Rico Rees, Kate Fetherston, Bill Yates, and Robert Smith kept me going with their love.

Todd Walton
Berkeley 1998